Aphasia Workbook
Foods - Book 1: Everyday Foods

By Florence Jones

This collection of books was created for my father who has Aphasia. Over the months while working with my father on his speech therapy homework, I realized how difficult it was for him to identify the hand-drawn black and white pictures that were presented to him on his worksheets.

In the beginning I remembered the doctor telling me to make every visit a productive visit. Having a tangible book that he can take with him and one that anyone can pick up and use added consistency to his recovery.

I tried workbooks made for children, however, these seemed to insult his intelligence. I also tried computer-based speech therapy applications which were only available when he had access to a computer. He seemed to progress faster when he worked one on one with another human being.

Each page includes photographs of different items common to every day living. Also on each page there are three levels of difficulty. How you choose to use each page is up to you and your patient or loved one. As I worked with my father to help him regain his speech, reading and writing, I realized the process was the same as for a child. First you learn to speak, then read, followed by writing. There are also different levels of Aphasia: one person may regain speaking very quickly while another not so quickly.

Get Started - There are three steps on each page:

Step 1 - Identify the picture: point to the picture and speak it out load. Have your patient or loved one repeat the word over and over, day after day. If your patient or loved one has severe Aphasia you might want to just do this step until your patient or loved one is able to identify the pictures. While working on this section you can reinforce the lesson by using the actual object in the picture.

Step 2 – Use the word in a sentence: this section is designed to help the patient identify the object in use. Each sentence has been chosen to help the patient regain basic sentences for every day use. Read the sentence and fill in the word. Have the patient or loved one try to verbally fill in the word own his own. He or she might need to be cued. While working on this section you can reinforce the lesson by using the actual objects.

Step 3 – Writing: after your patient or loved one has learned the objects the final step is writing the word. Have your patient write over the grayed out word, then encourage him or her to continue on their own.

Pasta

1. Point to the picture and say the word. Then have your patient repeat the word.

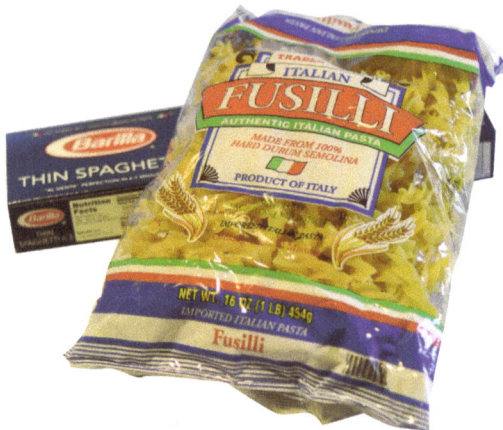

I like sauce on my _____ .

2. Read the sentence to your patient and verbally fill in the word. Read the sentence again and have your patient verbally fill in the missing word.

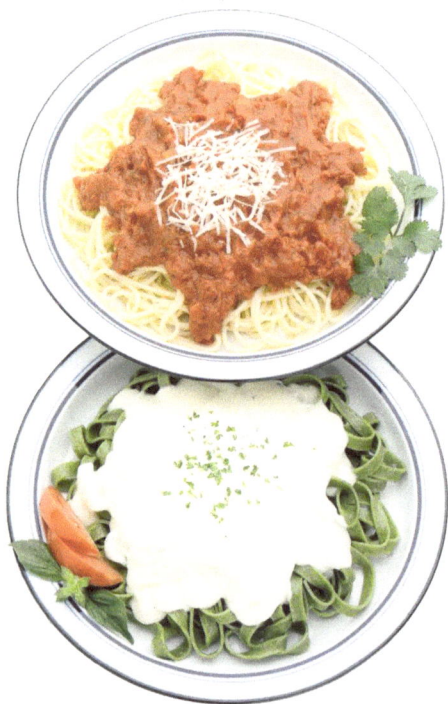

Aphasia Workbook, Foods - Book 1: Everyday Foods, Copyright 2013

3. Have your patient practice writing the word. Trace over each shaded word then repeat the word several times on each line.

Pasta

Pasta _____

Pasta _____

Pasta _____

Pasta _____

Pasta _____

Pasta _____

Pasta _____

Pasta _____

Pasta _____

Pasta _____

Pasta _____

Pasta _____

Pasta _____

Pasta _____

Pasta _____

Ceral

1. Point to the picture and say the word. Then have your patient repeat the word.

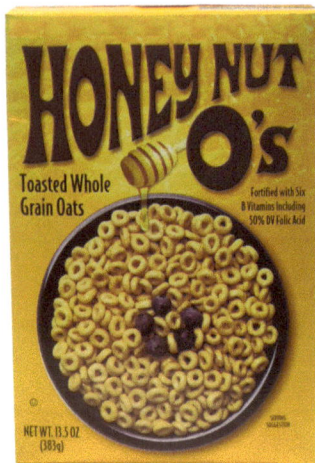

I would like bannas on my _____.

2. Read the sentence to your patient and verbally fill in the word. Read the sentence again and have your patient verbally fill in the missing word.

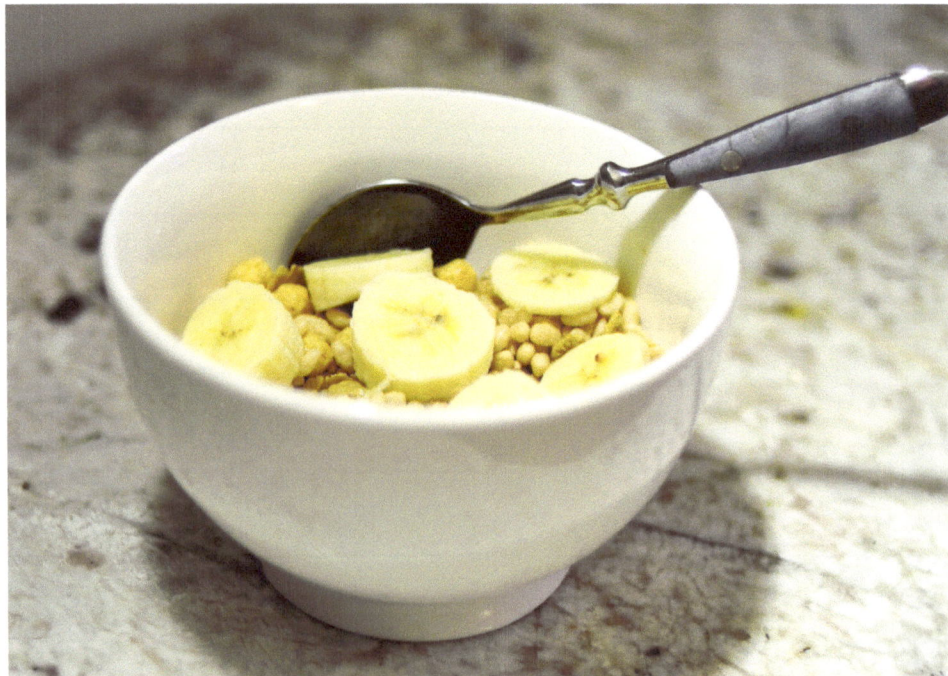

Aphasia Workbook, Foods - Book 1: Everyday Foods, Copyright 2013

3. Have your patient practice writing the word. Trace over each shaded word then repeat the word several times on each line..

Ceral

Ceral _____

Ceral _____

Ceral _____

Ceral _____

Ceral _____

Ceral _____

Ceral _____

Ceral _____

Ceral _____

Ceral _____

Ceral _____

Ceral _____

Ceral _____

Ceral _____

Ceral _____

Cookies

1. Point to the picture and say the word. Then have your patient repeat the word.

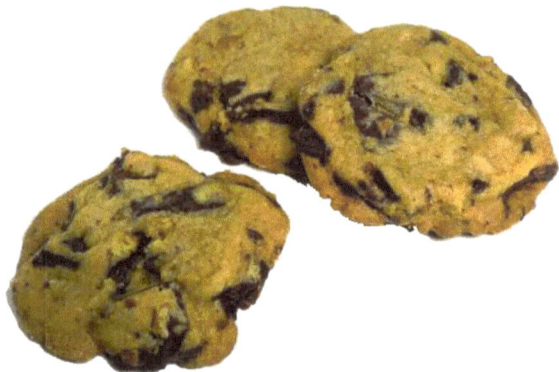

I like milk with my _____ .

2. Read the sentence to your patient and verbally fill in the word. Read the sentence again and have your patient verbally fill in the missing word.

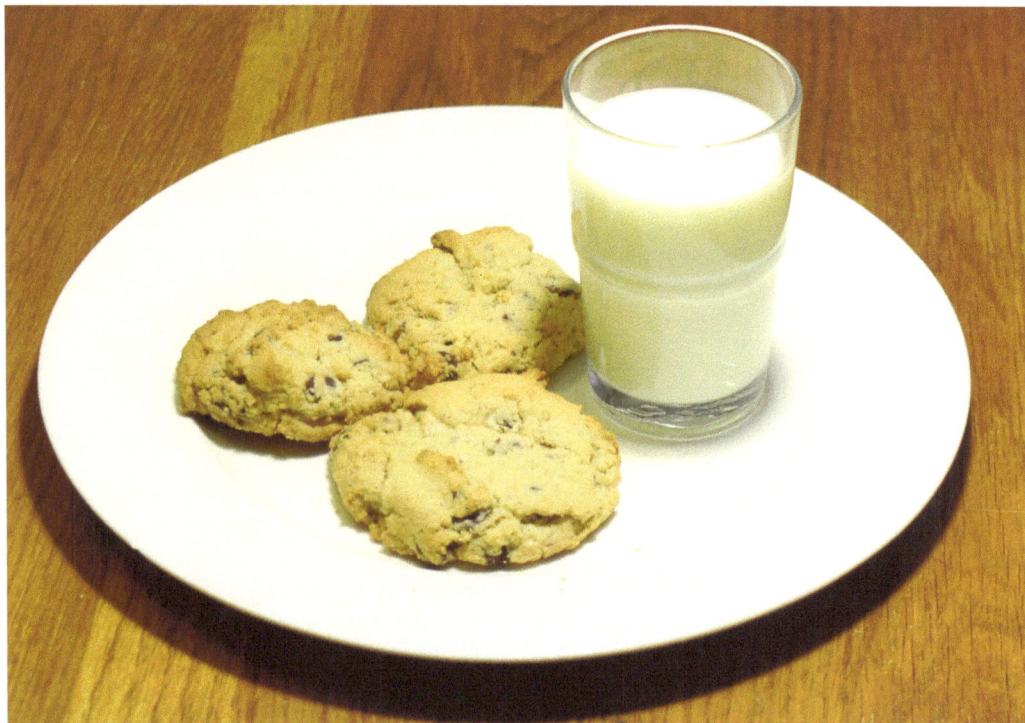

Aphasia Workbook, Foods - Book 1: Everyday Foods, Copyright 2013

3. Have your patient practice writing the word. Trace over each shaded word then repeat the word several times on each line.

Cookies

Cookies _____

Cookies _____

Cookies _____

Cookies _____

Cookies _____

Cookies _____

Cookies _____

Cookies _____

Cookies _____

Cookies _____

Cookies _____

Cookies _____

Cookies _____

Cookies _____

Cookies _____

Rice

1. Point to the picture and say the word. Then have your patient repeat the word.

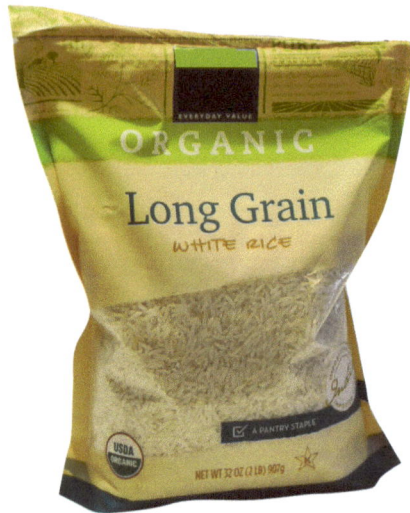

I like _____ with my beans.

2. Read the sentence to your patient and verbally fill in the word. Read the sentence again and have your patient verbally fill in the missing word.

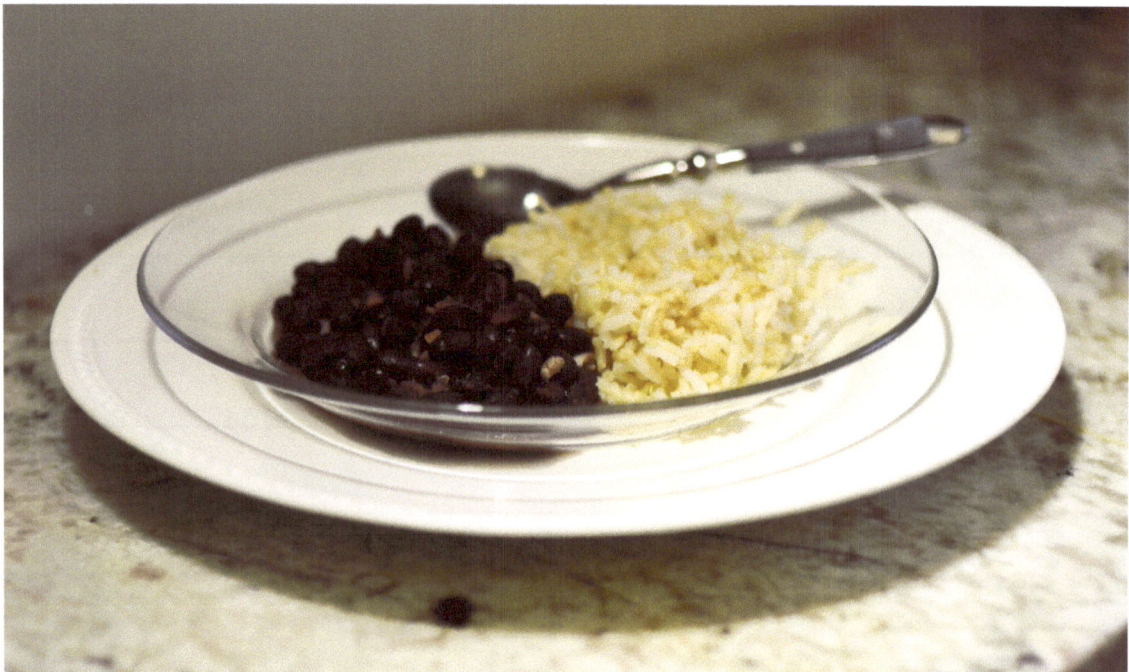

Aphasia Workbook, Foods - Book 1: Everyday Foods, Copyright 2013

3. Have your patient practice writing the word. Trace over each shaded word then repeat the word several times on each line.

Rice

Rice _____

Rice _____

Rice _____

Rice _____

Rice _____

Rice _____

Rice _____

Rice _____

Rice _____

Rice _____

Rice _____

Rice _____

Rice _____

Rice _____

Rice _____

Beans

1. Point to the picture and say the word. Then have your patient repeat the word.

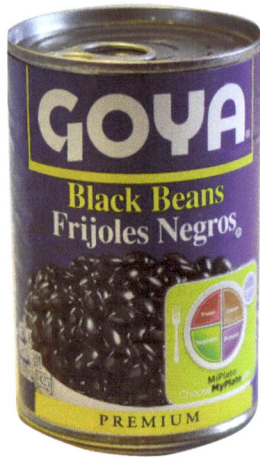

I like _____ with my rice.

2. Read the sentence to your patient and verbally fill in the word. Read the sentence again and have your patient verbally fill in the missing word.

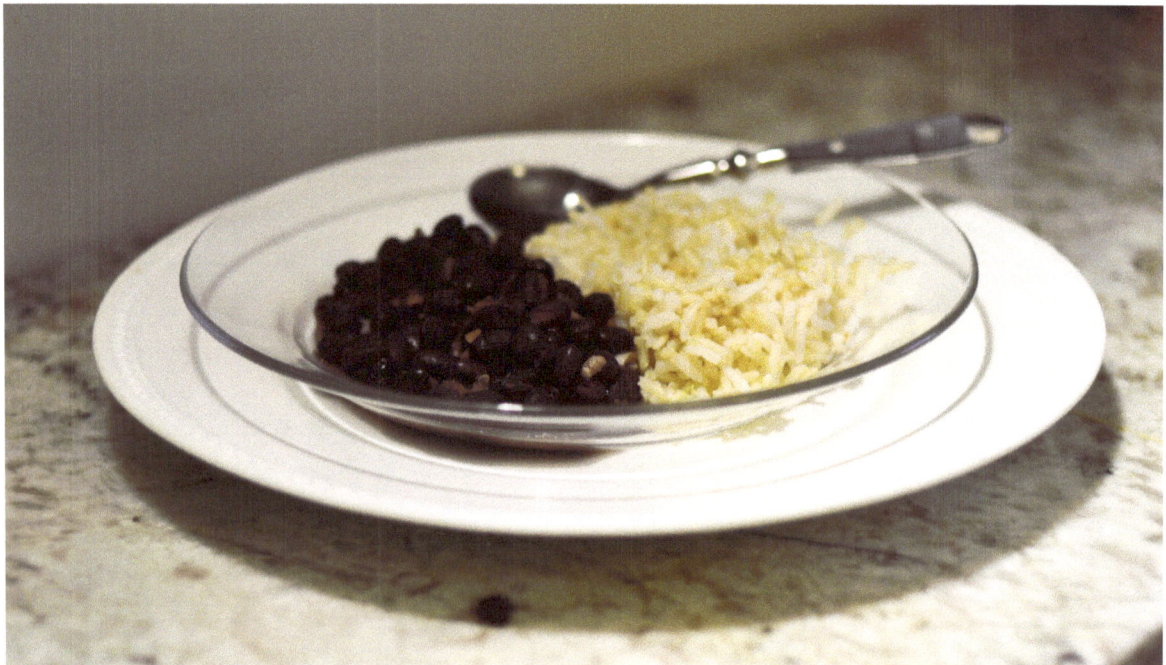

3. Have your patient practice writing the word. Trace over each shaded word then repeat the word several times on each line.

Beans

Beans _____

Beans _____

Beans _____

Beans _____

Beans _____

Beans _____

Beans _____

Beans _____

Beans _____

Beans _____

Beans _____

Beans _____

Beans _____

Beans _____

Beans _____

Fish

1. Point to the picture and say the word. Then have your patient repeat the word.

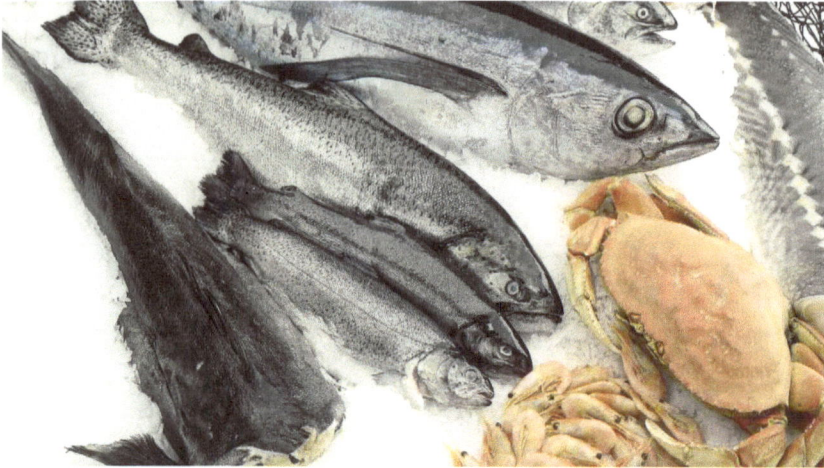

May I have _____, please.

2. Read the sentence to your patient and verbally fill in the word. Read the sentence again and have your patient verbally fill in the missing word.

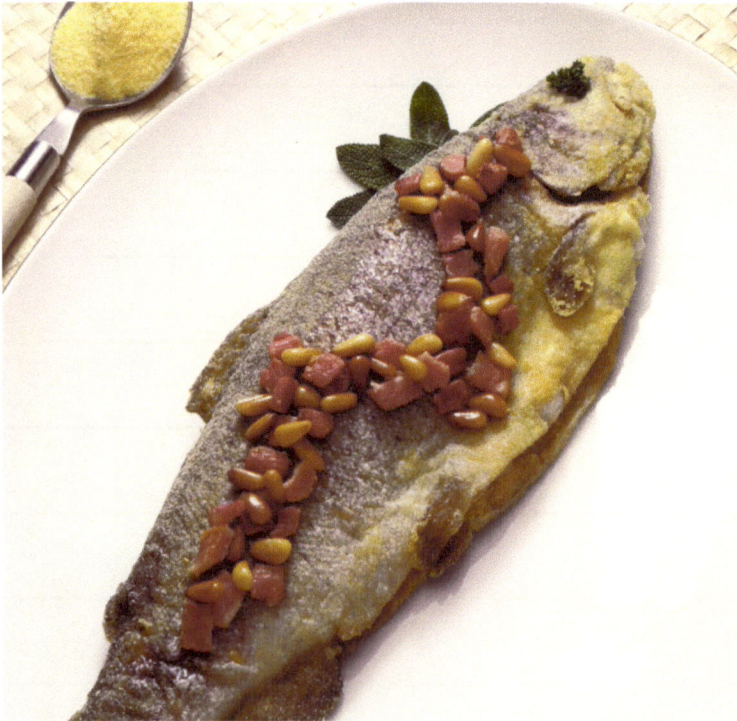

Aphasia Workbook, Foods - Book 1: Everyday Foods, Copyright 2013

3. Have your patient practice writing the word. Trace over each shaded word then repeat the word several times on each line.

Fish

Fish _____

Fish _____

Fish _____

Fish _____

Fish _____

Fish _____

Fish _____

Fish _____

Fish _____

Fish _____

Fish _____

Fish _____

Fish _____

Fish _____

Fish _____

Fish _____

Chicken

1. Point to the picture and say the word. Then have your patient repeat the word.

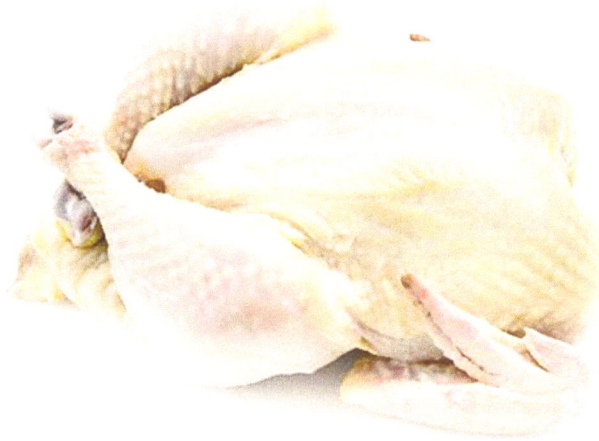

I would like roasted _____, please.

2. Read the sentence to your patient and verbally fill in the word. Read the sentence again and have your patient verbally fill in the missing word.

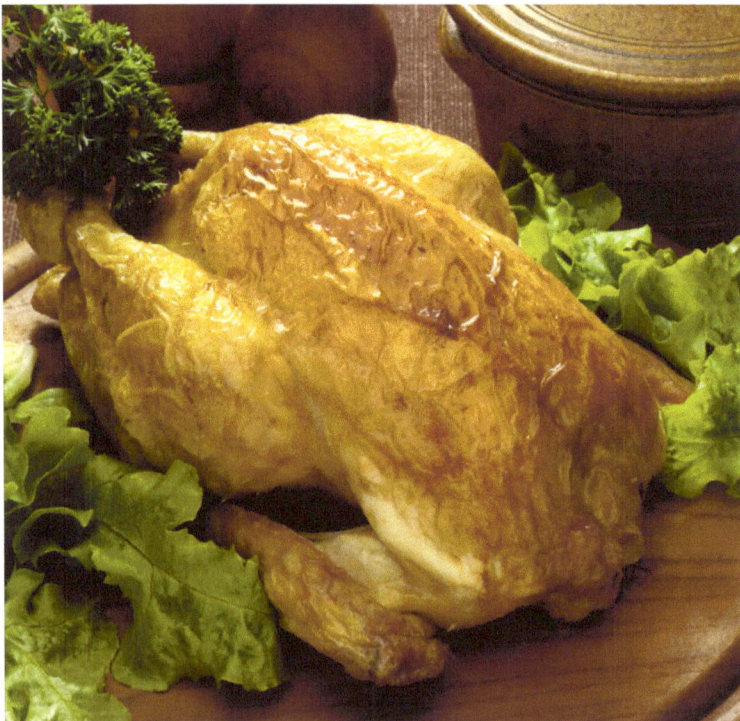

3. Have your patient practice writing the word. Trace over each shaded word then repeat the word several times on each line.

Chicken

Chicken _____

Chicken _____

Chicken _____

Chicken _____

Chicken _____

Chicken _____

Chicken _____

Chicken _____

Chicken _____

Chicken _____

Chicken _____

Chicken _____

Chicken _____

Chicken _____

Chicken _____

Beef

1. Point to the picture and say the word. Then have your patient repeat the word.

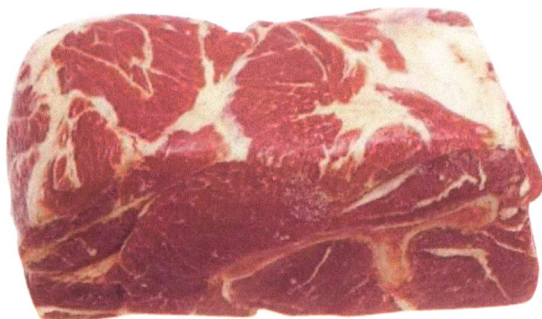

I would like a _____ for dinner, please.

2. Read the sentence to your patient and verbally fill in the word. Read the sentence again and have your patient verbally fill in the missing word.

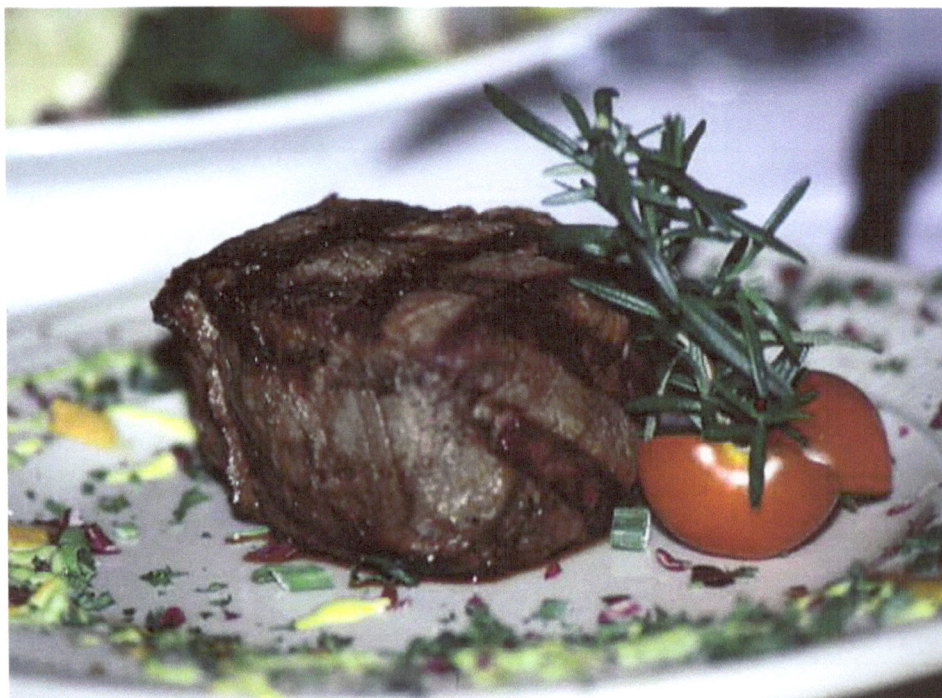

Aphasia Workbook, Foods - Book 1: Everyday Foods, Copyright 2013

3. Have your patient practice writing the word. Trace over each shaded word then repeat the word several times on each line.

Beef

Beef _____

Beef _____

Beef _____

Beef _____

Beef _____

Beef _____

Beef _____

Beef _____

Beef _____

Beef _____

Beef _____

Beef _____

Beef _____

Beef _____

Beef _____

Cabbage

1. Point to the picture and say the word. Then have your patient repeat the word.

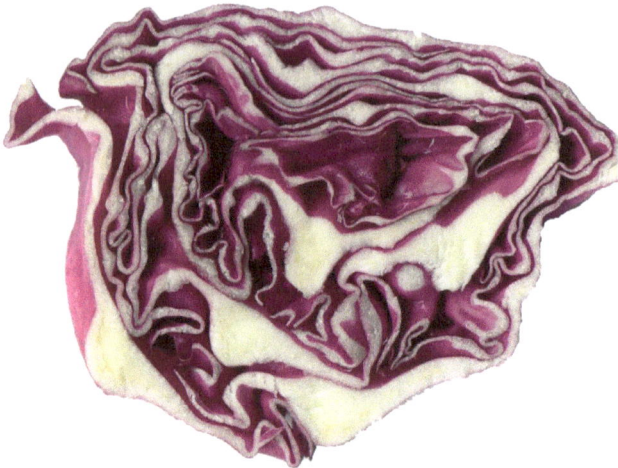

I would like _____with corn beef, please.

2. Read the sentence to your patient and verbally fill in the word. Read the sentence again and have your patient verbally fill in the missing word.

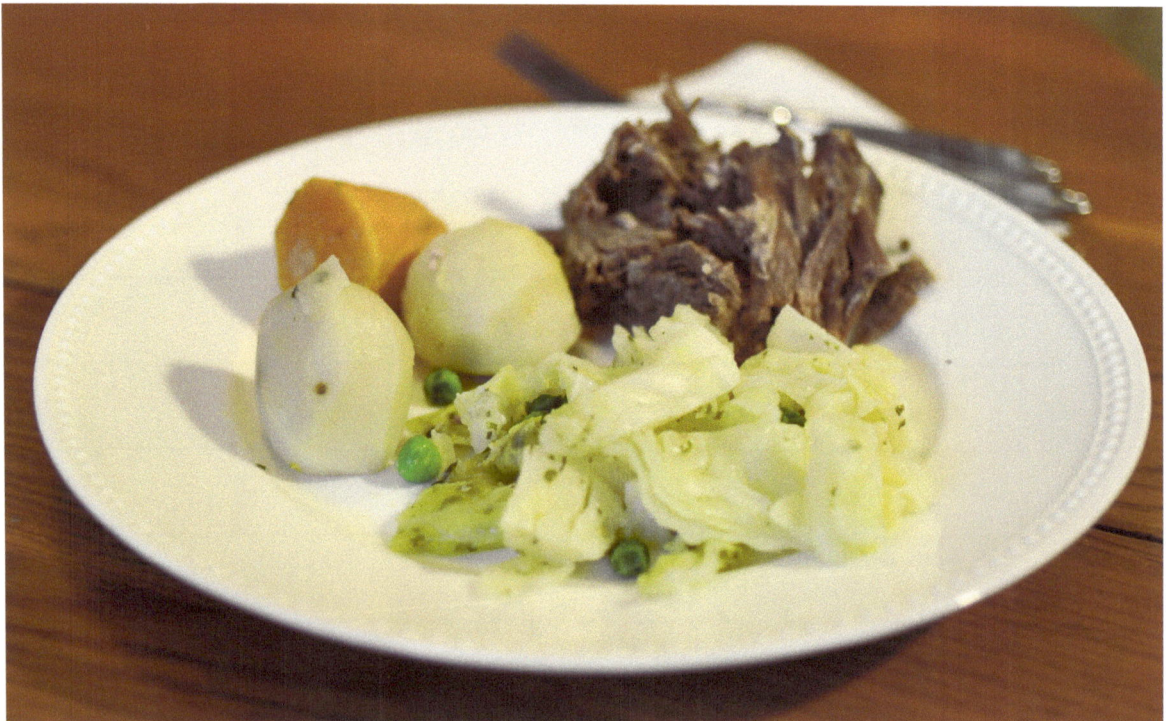

Aphasia Workbook, Foods - Book 1: Everyday Foods, Copyright 2013

3. Have your patient practice writing the word. Trace over each shaded word then repeat the word several times on each line.

Cabbage

Cabbage _____

Cabbage _____

Cabbage _____

Cabbage _____

Cabbage _____

Cabbage _____

Cabbage _____

Cabbage _____

Cabbage _____

Cabbage _____

Cabbage _____

Cabbage _____

Cabbage _____

Cabbage _____

Cabbage _____

Cabbage _____

Milk

1. Point to the picture and say the word. Then have your patient repeat the word.

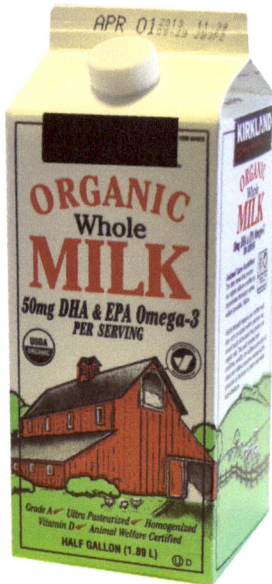

May I have a glass of _____.

2. Read the sentence to your patient and verbally fill in the word. Read the sentence again and have your patient verbally fill in the missing word.

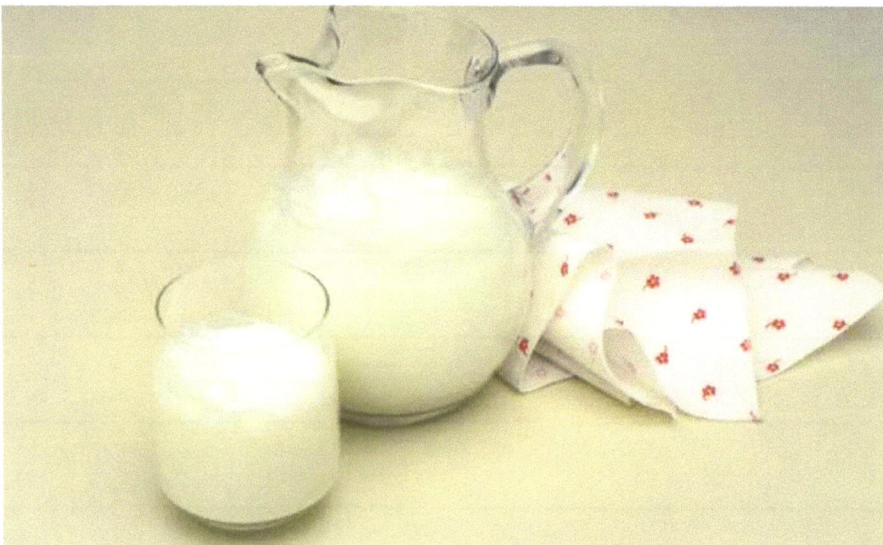

3. Have your patient practice writing the word. Trace over each shaded word then repeat the word several times on each line.

Milk

Milk _____

Milk _____

Milk _____

Milk _____

Milk _____

Milk _____

Milk _____

Milk _____

Milk _____

Milk _____

Milk _____

Milk _____

Milk _____

Milk _____

Milk _____

Milk _____

Salt + Pepper

1. Point to the picture and say the word. Then have your patient repeat the word.

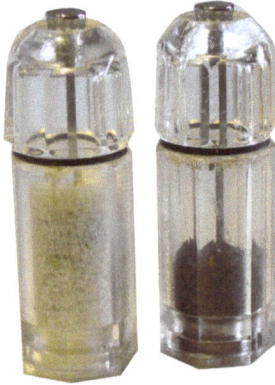

I put _____ and _____ on my food.

2. Read the sentence to your patient and verbally fill in the word. Read the sentence again and have your patient verbally fill in the missing word.

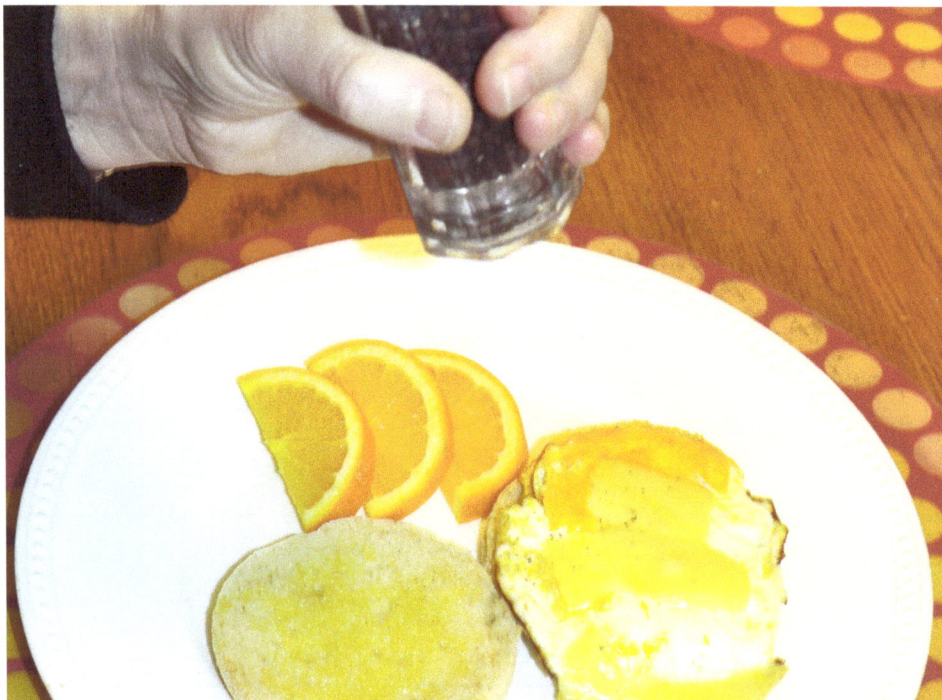

Aphasia Workbook, Foods - Book 1: Everyday Foods, Copyright 2013

3. Have your patient practice writing the word. Trace over each shaded word then repeat the word several times on each line.

Salt + Pepper

Salt + Pepper _____

Salt + Pepper _____

Salt + Pepper _____

Salt + Pepper _____

Salt + Pepper _____

Salt + Pepper _____

Salt + Pepper _____

Salt + Pepper _____

Salt + Pepper _____

Salt + Pepper _____

Salt + Pepper _____

Salt + Pepper _____

Salt + Pepper _____

Salt + Pepper _____

Salt + Pepper _____

Salt + Pepper _____

Coffee

1. Point to the picture and say the word. Then have your patient repeat the word.

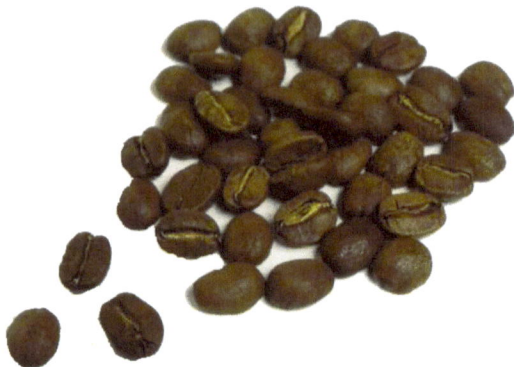

I like sugar for my _____ .

2. Read the sentence to your patient and verbally fill in the word. Read the sentence again and have your patient verbally fill in the missing word.

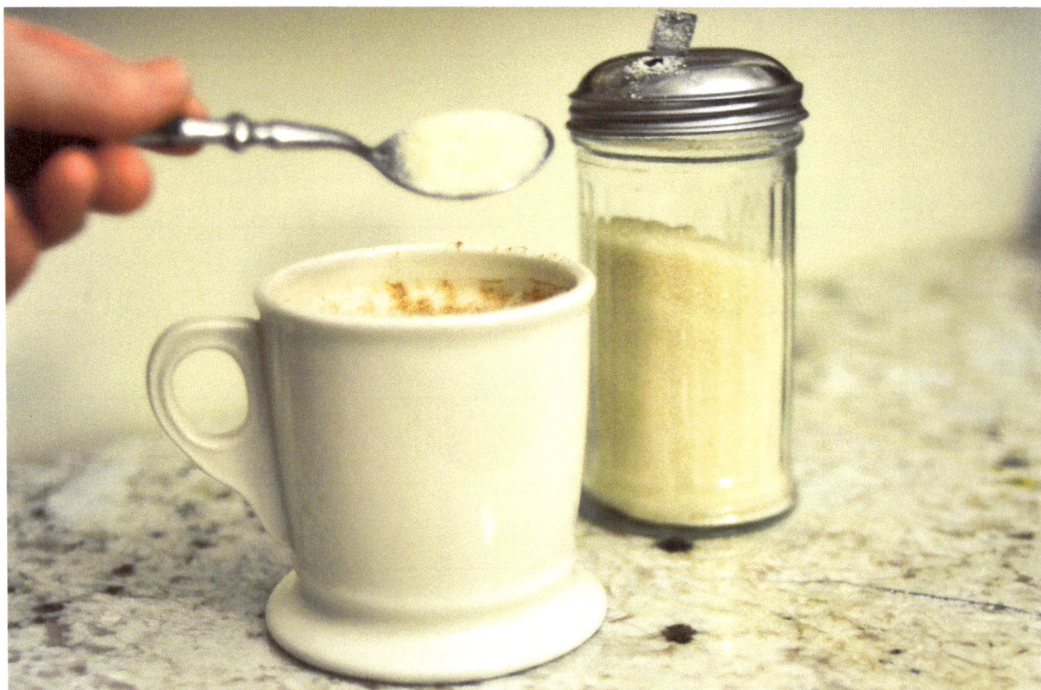

Aphasia Workbook, Foods - Book 1: Everyday Foods, Copyright 2013

3. Have your patient practice writing the word. Trace over each shaded word then repeat the word several times on each line.

Coffee

Coffee _____

Coffee _____

Coffee _____

Coffee _____

Coffee _____

Coffee _____

Coffee _____

Coffee _____

Coffee _____

Coffee _____

Coffee _____

Coffee _____

Coffee _____

Coffee _____

Coffee _____

Coffee _____

Tea

1. Point to the picture and say the word. Then have your patient repeat the word.

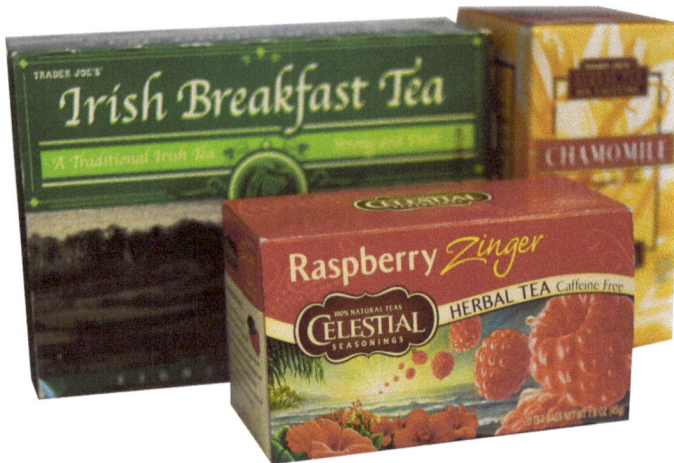

May I have a cup of black _____.

2. Read the sentence to your patient and verbally fill in the word. Read the sentence again and have your patient verbally fill in the missing word.

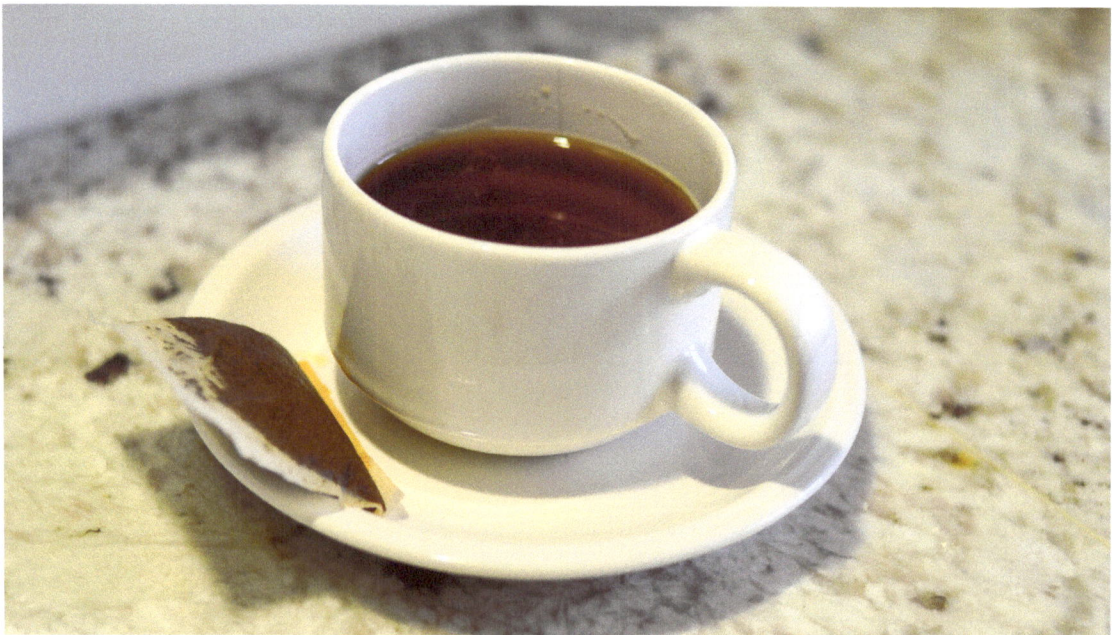

Aphasia Workbook, Foods - Book 1: Everyday Foods, Copyright 2013

3. Have your patient practice writing the word. Trace over each shaded word then repeat the word several times on each line.

Tea

Tea _____

Tea _____

Tea _____

Tea _____

Tea _____

Tea _____

Tea _____

Tea _____

Tea _____

Tea _____

Tea _____

Tea _____

Tea _____

Tea _____

Tea _____

Potato Chips

1. Point to the picture and say the word. Then have your patient repeat the word.

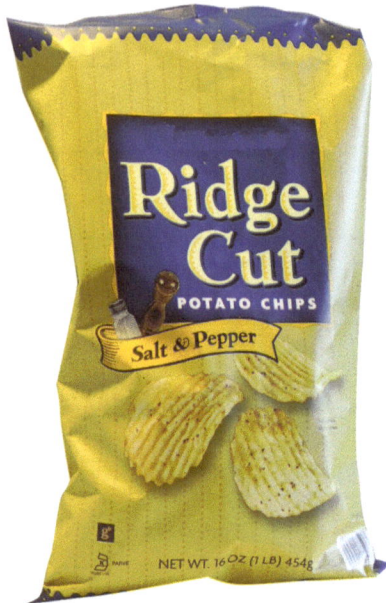

May I have some _____ , please.

2. Read the sentence to your patient and verbally fill in the word. Read the sentence again and have your patient verbally fill in the missing word.

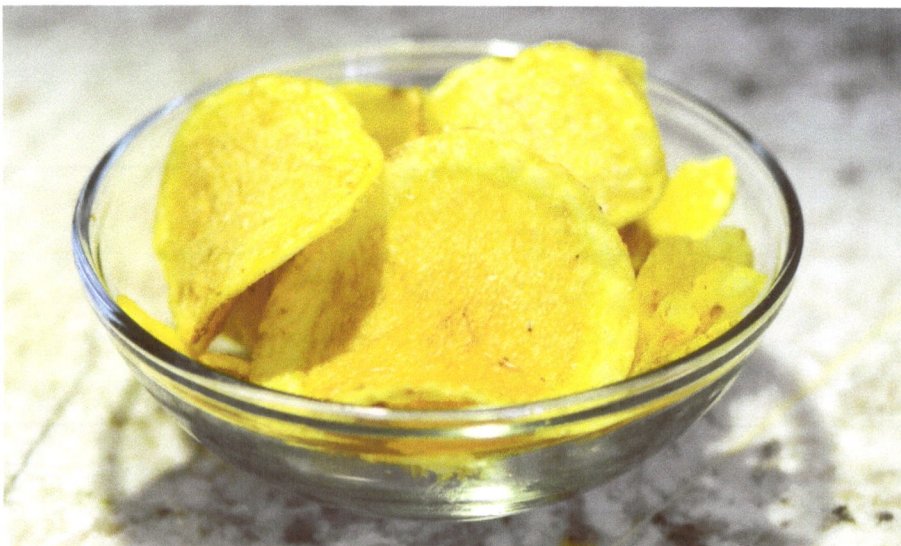

Aphasia Workbook, Foods - Book 1: Everyday Foods, Copyright 2013

3. Have your patient practice writing the word. Trace over each shaded word then repeat the word several times on each line.

Potato Chips

Potato Chips _____

Potato Chips _____

Potato Chips _____

Potato Chips _____

Potato Chips _____

Potato Chips _____

Potato Chips _____

Potato Chips _____

Potato Chips _____

Potato Chips _____

Potato Chips _____

Potato Chips _____

Potato Chips _____

Potato Chips _____

Potato Chips _____

Salad Dressing

1. Point to the picture and say the word. Then have your patient repeat the word.

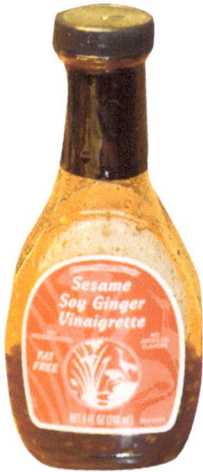

May I have _____ for my salad.

2. Read the sentence to your patient and verbally fill in the word. Read the sentence again and have your patient verbally fill in the missing word.

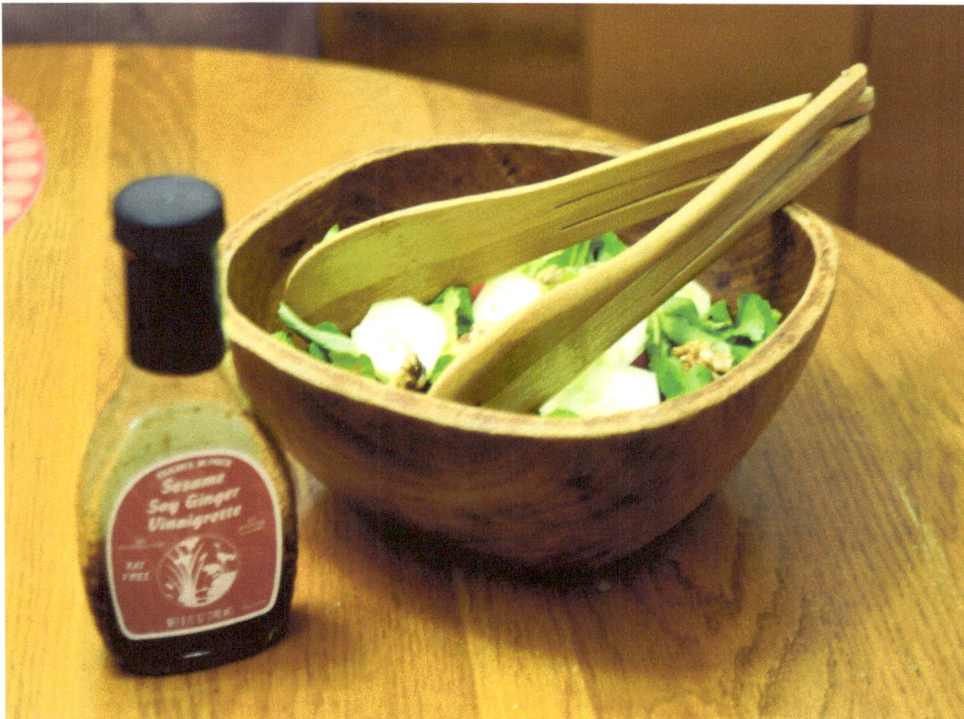

3. Have your patient practice writing the word. Trace over each shaded word then repeat the word several times on each line.

Salad Dressing

Salad Dressing_____

Salad Dressing_____

Salad Dressing_____

Salad Dressing_____

Salad Dressing_____

Salad Dressing_____

Salad Dressing_____

Salad Dressing_____

Salad Dressing_____

Salad Dressing_____

Salad Dressing_____

Salad Dressing_____

Salad Dressing_____

Salad Dressing_____

Salad Dressing_____

Salad Dressing_____

Ketchup

1. Point to the picture and say the word. Then have your patient repeat the word.

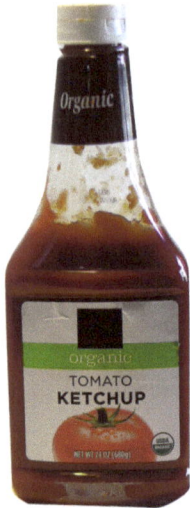

I like _____ and mustard on my hotdog.

2. Read the sentence to your patient and verbally fill in the word. Read the sentence again and have your patient verbally fill in the missing word.

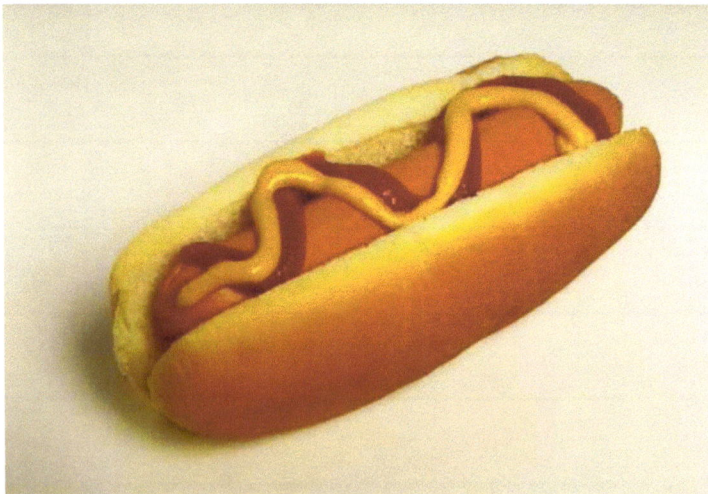

3. Have your patient practice writing the word. Trace over each shaded word then repeat the word several times on each line.

Ketchup

Ketchup _____

Ketchup _____

Ketchup _____

Ketchup _____

Ketchup _____

Ketchup _____

Ketchup _____

Ketchup _____

Ketchup _____

Ketchup _____

Ketchup _____

Ketchup _____

Ketchup _____

Ketchup _____

Ketchup _____

Ketchup _____

Mustard

1. Point to the picture and say the word. Then have your patient repeat the word.

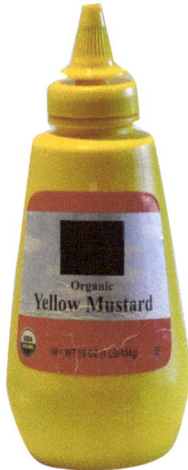

I like _____ and Ketcup on my hot dog.

2. Read the sentence to your patient and verbally fill in the word. Read the sentence again and have your patient verbally fill in the missing word.

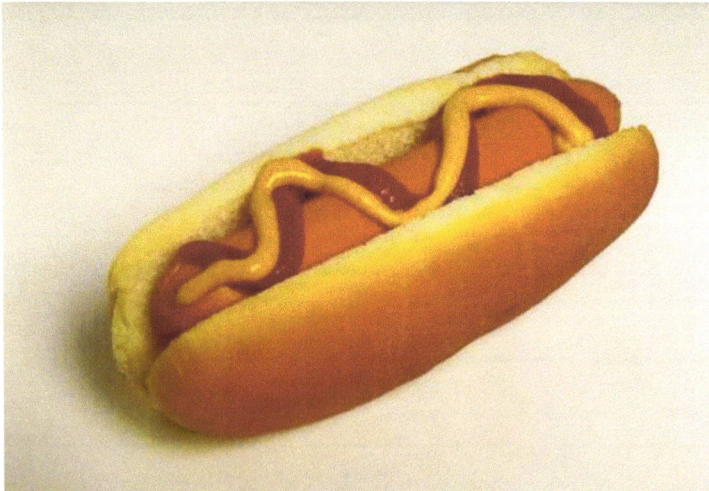

3. Have your patient practice writing the word. Trace over each shaded word then repeat the word several times on each line.

Mustard

Mustard_____

Mustard_____

Mustard_____

Mustard_____

Mustard_____

Mustard_____

Mustard_____

Mustard_____

Mustard_____

Mustard_____

Mustard_____

Mustard_____

Mustard_____

Mustard_____

Mustard_____

Mustard_____

Mayonnaise

1. Point to the picture and say the word. Then have your patient repeat the word.

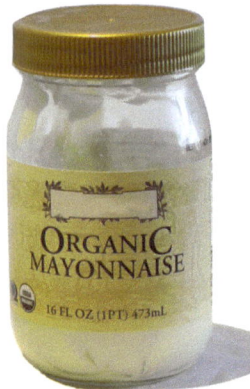

I would like _____ on my sandwich, please.

2. Read the sentence to your patient and verbally fill in the word. Read the sentence again and have your patient verbally fill in the missing word.

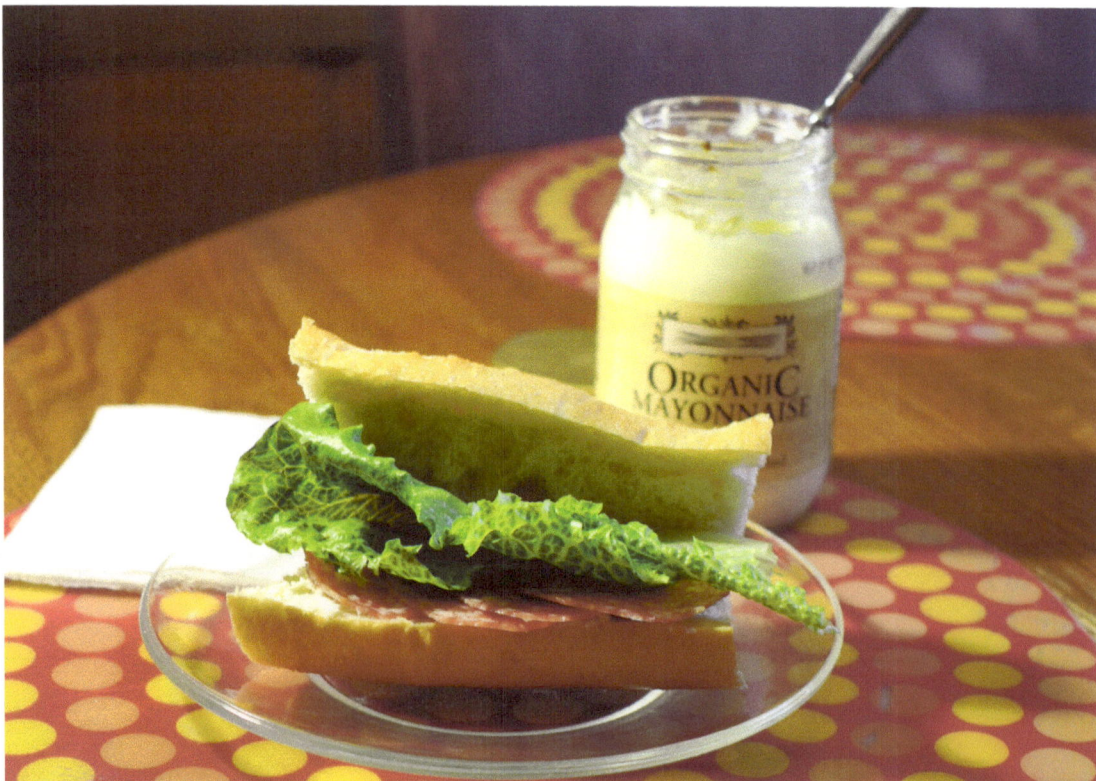

3. Have your patient practice writing the word. Trace over each shaded word then repeat the word several times on each line.

Mayonnaise

Mayonnaise _____

Mayonnaise _____

Mayonnaise _____

Mayonnaise _____

Mayonnaise _____

Mayonnaise _____

Mayonnaise _____

Mayonnaise _____

Mayonnaise _____

Mayonnaise _____

Mayonnaise _____

Mayonnaise _____

Mayonnaise _____

Mayonnaise _____

Mayonnaise _____

Mayonnaise _____

Yogurt

1. Point to the picture and say the word. Then have your patient repeat the word.

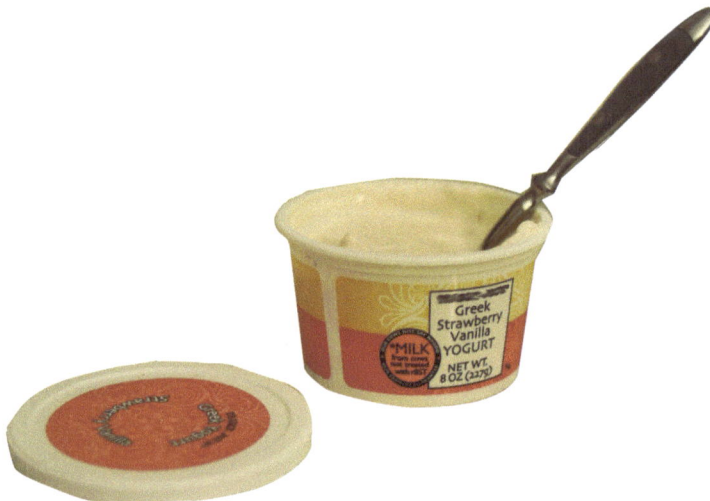

I like a _____on fruit salad.

2. Read the sentence to your patient and verbally fill in the word. Read the sentence again and have your patient verbally fill in the missing word.

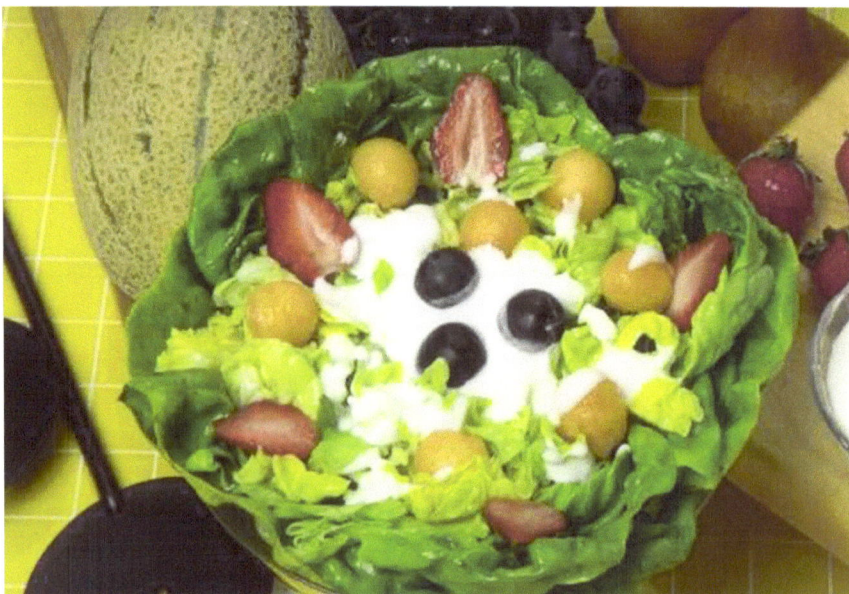

3. Have your patient practice writing the word. Trace over each shaded word then repeat the word several times on each line.

Yogurt

Yogurt_____

Yogurt_____

Yogurt_____

Yogurt_____

Yogurt_____

Yogurt_____

Yogurt_____

Yogurt_____

Yogurt_____

Yogurt_____

Yogurt_____

Yogurt_____

Yogurt_____

Yogurt_____

Yogurt_____

Cheese

1. Point to the picture and say the word. Then have your patient repeat the word.

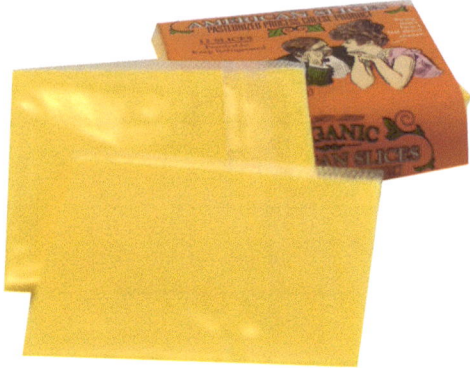

May I have a slice of _____on my burger.

2. Read the sentence to your patient and verbally fill in the word. Read the sentence again and have your patient verbally fill in the missing word.

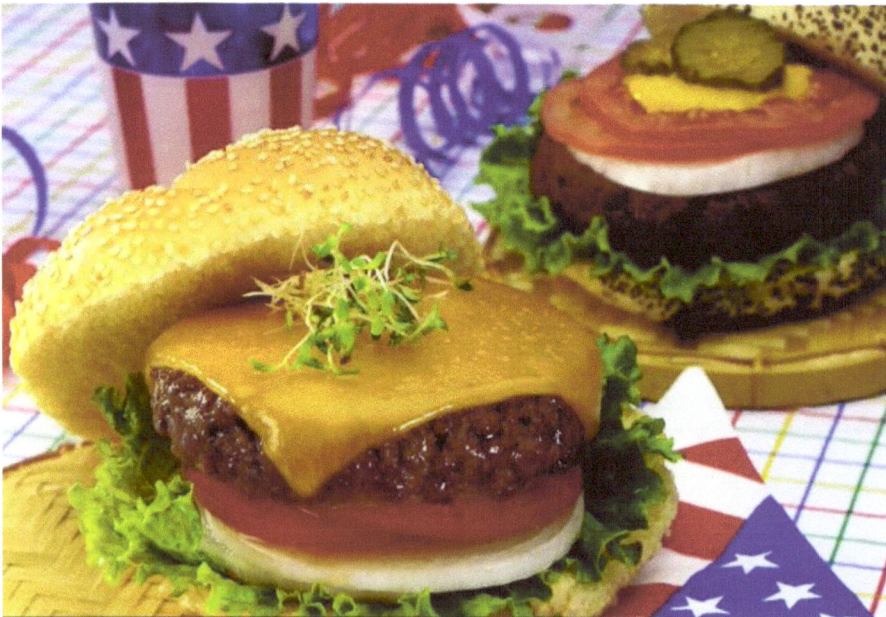

3. Have your patient practice writing the word. Trace over each shaded word then repeat the word several times on each line.

Cheese

Cheese _____

Cheese _____

Cheese _____

Cheese _____

Cheese _____

Cheese _____

Cheese _____

Cheese _____

Cheese _____

Cheese _____

Cheese _____

Cheese _____

Cheese _____

Cheese _____

Cheese _____

Cheese _____

Jam

1. Point to the picture and say the word. Then have your patient repeat the word.

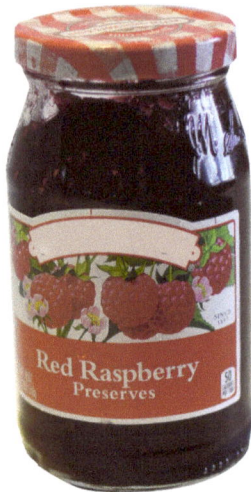

May I have _____ for my toast, please.

2. Read the sentence to your patient and verbally fill in the word. Read the sentence again and have your patient verbally fill in the missing word.

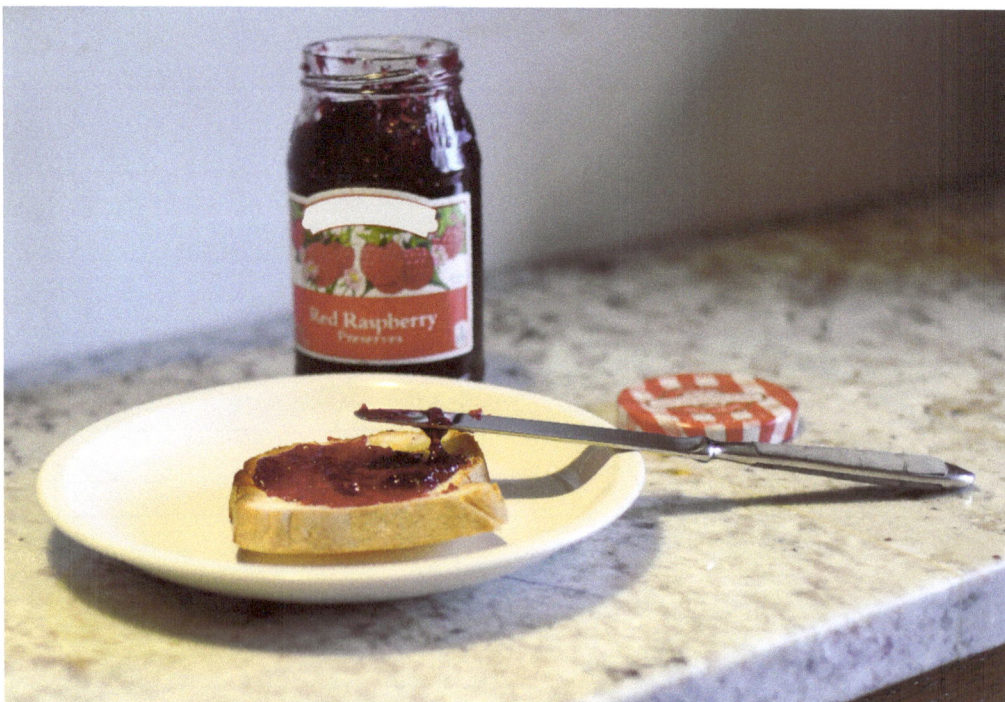

Aphasia Workbook, Foods - Book 1: Everyday Foods, Copyright 2013

3. Have your patient practice writing the word. Trace over each shaded word then repeat the word several times on each line.

Jam

Jam _____

Jam _____

Jam _____

Jam _____

Jam _____

Jam _____

Jam _____

Jam _____

Jam _____

Jam _____

Jam _____

Jam _____

Jam _____

Jam _____

Jam _____

Bread

1. Point to the picture and say the word. Then have your patient repeat the word.

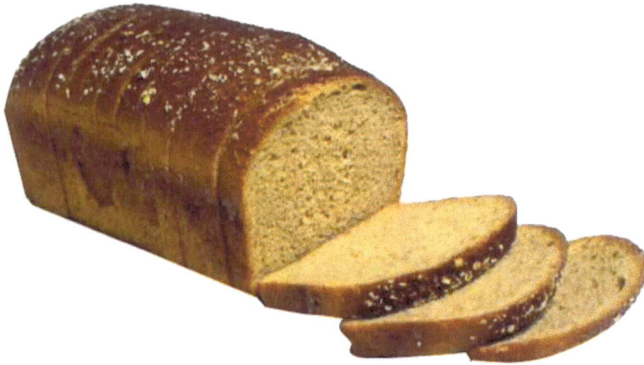

Would you toast my_____, please.

2. Read the sentence to your patient and verbally fill in the word. Read the sentence again and have your patient verbally fill in the missing word.

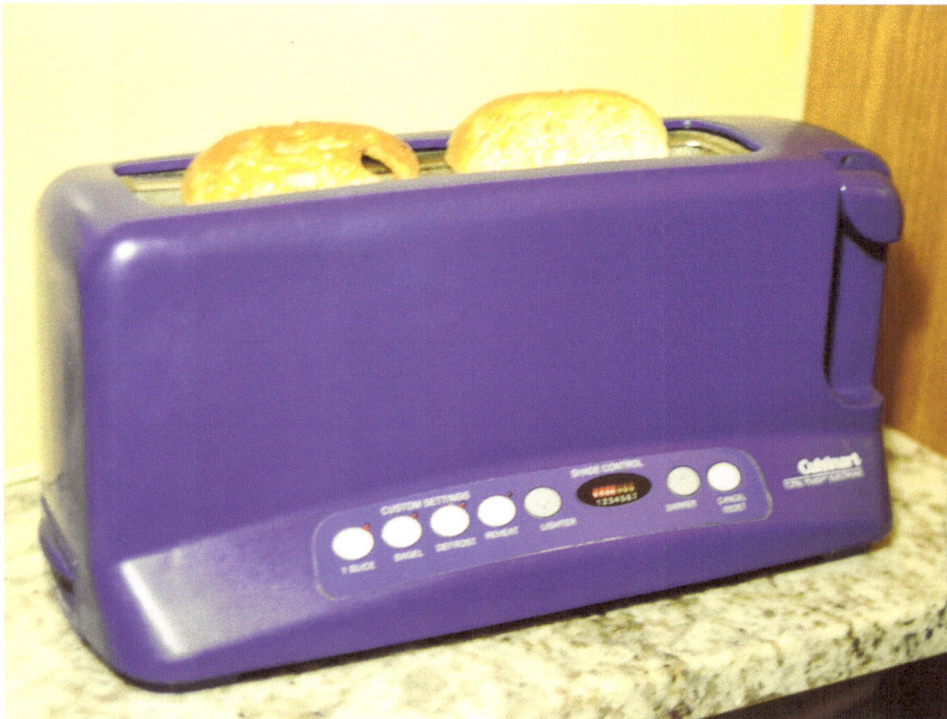

Aphasia Workbook, Foods - Book 1: Everyday Foods, Copyright 2013

3. Have your patient practice writing the word. Trace over each shaded word then repeat the word several times on each line.

Bread

Bread _____

Bread _____

Bread _____

Bread _____

Bread _____

Bread _____

Bread _____

Bread _____

Bread _____

Bread _____

Bread _____

Bread _____

Bread _____

Bread _____

Bread _____

Eggs

1. Point to the picture and say the word. Then have your patient repeat the word.

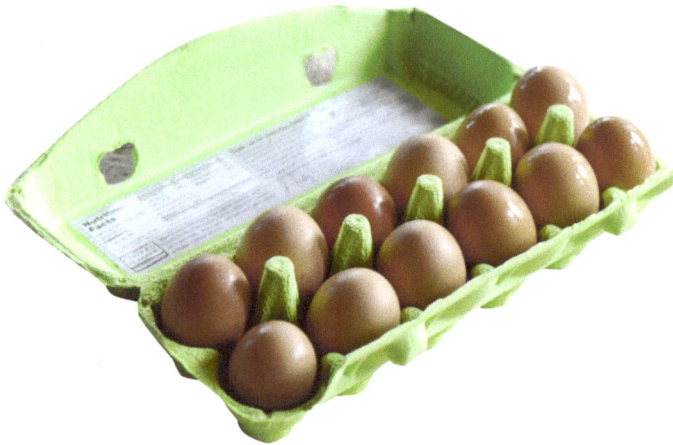

I like my _____ scrabbled/fried/poached.

2. Read the sentence to your patient and verbally fill in the word. Read the sentence again and have your patient verbally fill in the missing word.

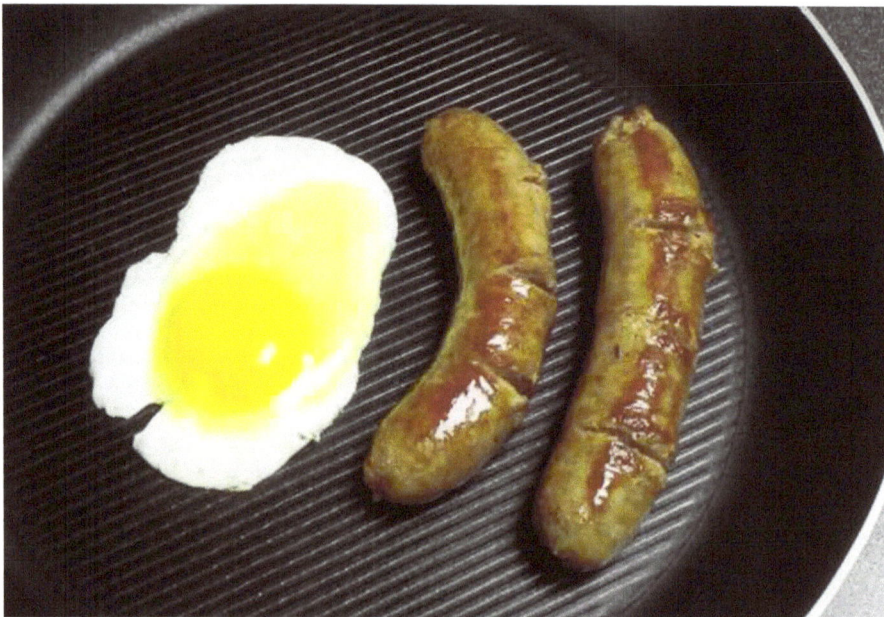

Aphasia Workbook, Foods - Book 1: Everyday Foods, Copyright 2013

3. Have your patient practice writing the word. Trace over each shaded word then repeat the word several times on each line.

Eggs

Eggs _____

Eggs _____

Eggs _____

Eggs _____

Eggs _____

Eggs _____

Eggs _____

Eggs _____

Eggs _____

Eggs _____

Eggs _____

Eggs _____

Eggs _____

Eggs _____

Eggs _____

Eggs _____

Dedicated to my father
David Jones

This series of Aphasia Workbooks is available for purchase at
www.amazon.com or www.createspace.com (for larger quantities)